The Gift Of Healthy Aging: A Guide To Living An Active, Long And Fulfilling Life

DISCLAIMER

The information contained in this resource is general in nature and for informative purposes only.

The Author assumes no responsibility whatsoever, under any circumstances, for any actions taken as a result of the information contained herein.

You are required to seek professional help if needed.

Before this document is duplicated or reproduced in any manner, the publisher's consent must be gained. Therefore, the contents within can neither be stored electronically, transferred, nor kept in a database.

Neither in Part nor full can the document be copied, scanned, faxed, or retained without approval from the publisher or creator.

Preface

A Spark to Ignite Your Golden Years

Have you ever looked in the mirror and realized you've reached an exciting new chapter in your life? A chapter brimming with possibilities, wisdom, and the freedom to pursue your passions? This book isn't about slowing down; it's about embracing the vibrant adventure that is healthy aging.

Perhaps you have questions. How can I stay active and independent? How can I manage stress and cultivate resilience? How can I secure my financial future and plan for a comfortable retirement? How can I stay connected and engaged in my community?

This book is your roadmap to a fulfilling golden age. Packed with practical tips, insightful strategies, and inspiring stories, it will empower you to take charge of your health, well-being, and happiness. We'll explore:

- **Finding Purpose and Passion**: Reignite your spark and discover activities that bring you joy and fulfillment.
- **Managing Stress and Cultivating Resilience**: Develop strategies to navigate life's challenges with greater ease and inner strength.
- **Financial Planning for the Future**: Build a secure financial foundation for a worry-free and independent future.
- **Creating a Safe and Supportive Home**: Modify your living space to enhance your safety and comfort, allowing you to age in place with confidence.

- **Senior Living Options**: Explore a variety of senior living arrangements to find the perfect fit for your needs and preferences.
- **Technology for a Connected Life**: Embrace user-friendly tools and resources that can simplify daily tasks, enhance your well-being, and keep you connected.
- **Advocacy and Community Resources**: Learn how to advocate for your rights, access valuable community services, and remain actively engaged in your community.

Throughout this journey, remember, you are not alone. This book is your companion, offering guidance, support, and inspiration as you embark on this exciting new chapter. So, turn the page, unlock the potential within you, and get ready to make the most of the incredible gift of aging!

Leo Chambers

Contents

Part 1: Embracing the Journey

Preface
- Introduction - Reframing Aging as a Positive Process

Introduction

Reframing Aging as a Positive Process

Imagine yourself standing on a mountain peak. Behind you stretches the path you've climbed, a journey filled with triumphs and challenges, breathtaking vistas and shadowed valleys. Before you lies a vast, uncharted landscape, bathed in the golden light of the setting sun. This, my friend, is aging. It's not the descent into a diminished state, but the ascent to a new and exciting plateau.

For generations, the narrative surrounding aging has been steeped in negativity. We've been bombarded with images of stooped figures and fading memories, a future filled with decline and limitations. But what if we reframed this narrative? What if aging wasn't just about the number of candles on your cake, but rather a vibrant chapter brimming with untapped potential?

This book is your guide to unlocking this potential. We'll embark on a journey together, exploring the science behind aging, debunking common myths, and discovering the pillars of well-being that will empower you to thrive in your golden years.

The Silver Lining: Why Aging is a Gift

Let's face it, the notion of getting older can be daunting. The thought of physical changes, diminishing eyesight, or the potential for chronic illness can instill a sense of apprehension. But before we succumb to fear, let's shift our perspective. Here's why aging is truly a gift:

- **Wisdom Gained**: Life experiences have etched invaluable lessons onto your soul. You've navigated love and loss, built careers, and raised families. This wealth of experience translates into wisdom, a potent tool for navigating life's complexities.
- **Greater Self-Awareness**: You've spent a lifetime learning who you are, what you value, and what truly matters. This self-awareness allows you to prioritize your well-being, pursue passions long neglected, and shed societal pressures that may have burdened you in your younger years.

- **Time to Pursue Passions**: With work commitments potentially lessened, you have the freedom to delve into long-held dreams. Write that novel, paint that masterpiece, master that musical instrument – the possibilities are endless.
- **Stronger Bonds**: Relationships forged in the fire of time deepen with age. You cherish loved ones with an even greater appreciation, valuing the connections that bring joy and comfort.
- **Gratitude for the Simple Things**: A sunrise, a cup of coffee, the laughter of loved ones – these simple pleasures take on a new meaning with age. You find joy in the everyday, appreciating life's small wonders.

The Myth Busters: Redefining Aging

Aging is not a one-size-fits-all process. Some individuals experience a natural decline in physical abilities at a slower pace, while others may face more challenges. Here are some common myths about aging that we need to debunk:

- **Myth 1: Aging means decline.** Absolutely not! While some physical changes are inevitable, a healthy lifestyle can significantly improve and maintain physical and cognitive function.

- **Myth 2: You can't learn new things when you're older.** Our brains have a remarkable ability to adapt and grow throughout our lives. Learning new skills keeps the mind sharp and can even help prevent cognitive decline.
- **Myth 3: Senior years are a time for isolation.** Social connection is crucial at any age, and even more so as we age. Strong social bonds can significantly improve physical and mental well-being.
- **Myth 4: A fulfilling life is a thing of the past.** On the contrary! With more free time and a wealth of experience, you have the opportunity to create a life brimming with purpose and passion.

A Journey of Empowerment: Embracing Your New Chapter

This book is your roadmap to a vibrant and fulfilling future. Here's what you can expect:

- **Science-backed strategies** to optimize your health, both physically and mentally.

- **Practical tips** for maintaining a healthy lifestyle, including nutrition, exercise, and sleep habits.
- **Guidance** on preventive healthcare and early detection strategies for age-related conditions.
- **Strategies** for staying socially connected, finding purpose, and managing stress.
- **Resources** to help you navigate the senior living landscape and access available support systems.

Aging is not a destination, but rather a continuation of your remarkable journey. It's a call to action, an opportunity to discover your best self and embrace the incredible potential that lies within. So, turn the page, my friend, and let's embark on this adventure together.

Chapter 1

The Science of Aging - Understanding the Biological Changes

As we embark on this journey of healthy aging, it's crucial to understand the biological changes that occur within our bodies. While the aging process is complex and not fully understood, scientists have identified several key factors at play:

Cellular Decline: The Hallmarks of Aging

Our bodies are composed of trillions of cells, the building blocks of life. These cells carry out essential functions, dividing and replicating to keep our tissues and organs functioning properly. However, with age, several cellular changes contribute to the aging process:

• Telomere Shortening: At the tips of each chromosome lies a structure called a telomere. These telomeres act like protective caps, safeguarding the integrity of our genetic information. Unfortunately, with each cell division, telomeres become progressively shorter. Once they reach a critical length, cells can no longer divide effectively, leading to tissue decline.

•   DNA Damage: Throughout our lives, our DNA is constantly bombarded by damaging agents like free radicals and ultraviolet radiation. While our bodies have repair mechanisms in place, their efficacy diminishes with age, leading to the accumulation of DNA damage, which can disrupt cellular function.

•   Epigenetic Changes: Epigenetics refers to the chemical modifications that influence gene expression without altering the DNA sequence itself. These epigenetic changes can become dysregulated with age, leading to the inappropriate activation or silencing of genes, ultimately impacting cellular function.

Cellular Senescence: When Cells Refuse to Retire

Some cells, upon encountering DNA damage or telomere shortening, enter a state of cellular senescence. These senescent cells remain alive but stop dividing. While this may seem like a good thing, preventing uncontrolled cell growth, it has a downside. Senescent cells secrete harmful substances called SASP (Senescence-Associated Secretory Phenotype) that can damage neighboring cells and contribute to chronic inflammation, a hallmark of many age-related diseases.

The Mitochondrial Theory of Aging: The Powerhouse Under Siege

Mitochondria are often referred to as the powerhouses of the cell, responsible for generating energy through a process called cellular respiration. Unfortunately, mitochondria also produce free radicals as a byproduct. With age, the number and function of mitochondria decline, leading to a decrease in energy production and a simultaneous increase in free radical damage. This vicious cycle contributes to cellular dysfunction and tissue decline.

The Hormonal Shift: A Delicate Balance

Hormones act as chemical messengers, regulating various bodily functions. As we age, our hormonal profile changes. Levels of sex hormones like estrogen, testosterone, and progesterone begin to decline. This hormonal shift can contribute to a variety of age-related changes, including decreased bone density, muscle loss, and changes in mood.

The Inflammatory Response: A Double-Edged Sword

Inflammation is a natural response to injury or infection. It's the body's attempt to heal and repair itself. However, chronic, low-grade inflammation is associated with various age-related diseases like heart disease, diabetes, and Alzheimer's. This chronic inflammation can be triggered by various factors, including cellular senescence, a dysfunctional immune system, and an unhealthy lifestyle.

Understanding Doesn't Mean Accepting: Strategies to Mitigate the Effects of Aging

While the science of aging paints a picture of cellular decline, it's important to remember that these processes are not inevitable. Many lifestyle modifications and interventions can significantly mitigate the effects of aging and promote healthy longevity:

• 	Healthy Diet: A diet rich in fruits, vegetables, whole grains, and lean protein provides essential nutrients to support cellular health and reduce inflammation.

•   Regular Exercise: Physical activity has been shown to improve mitochondrial function, reduce chronic inflammation, and promote cognitive function.

•   Quality Sleep: Sleep allows the body to repair and rejuvenate itself. Aim for 7-8 hours of quality sleep each night.

•   Stress Management: Chronic stress can exacerbate inflammation and accelerate cellular decline. Techniques like meditation and yoga can help manage stress effectively.

•   Supplements: Certain supplements like antioxidants and vitamin D may be beneficial in reducing oxidative damage and supporting overall health. However, consult your doctor before starting any supplements.

The Future of Aging Research: A Glimpse of Hope

The field of aging research is experiencing a revolution. Scientists are exploring various avenues to promote healthy longevity, including:

•   Telomere Lengthening: Research is underway to develop therapies that could potentially slow or reverse telomere shortening.

•   Senolytic Drugs: These drugs target senescent cells, aiming to clear them from the body and reduce their detrimental effects.

•   Hormone Replacement Therapy: While HRT has its limitations and potential risks, it can be beneficial for some individuals in managing symptoms associated with hormonal decline.

•   Personalized Medicine: This approach tailors interventions to an individual's unique genetic makeup and health profile. By understanding your specific risk factors and vulnerabilities, scientists can develop targeted therapies to promote healthy aging for you.

Beyond the Cell: The Impact of Lifestyle on Aging

The science of aging goes beyond the cellular level. Our lifestyle choices profoundly impact the rate at which we age and the quality of our later years. Here are some key areas to consider:

• 	Diet: As mentioned earlier, a healthy diet rich in fruits, vegetables, whole grains, and lean protein is crucial. Limiting processed foods, added sugars, and unhealthy fats can significantly reduce inflammation and promote cellular health.

• 	Exercise: Regular physical activity, including both cardio and strength training, is essential for maintaining muscle mass, improving bone density, and enhancing cognitive function. Aim for at least 30 minutes of moderate-intensity exercise most days of the week.

• 	Sleep: Chronic sleep deprivation disrupts hormonal balance, weakens the immune system, and contributes to cognitive decline. Prioritize sleep hygiene practices to ensure restful nights.

• 	Stress Management: Chronic stress triggers the release of cortisol, a hormone that can exacerbate inflammation and damage cells. Finding healthy ways to manage stress, such as meditation, yoga, or spending time in nature, is crucial for healthy aging.

• 	Social Connection: Strong social bonds have been shown to improve both physical and mental well-being. Nurture your relationships with friends and family, and consider joining social groups or volunteering in your community.

•   Mental Stimulation: Keeping your mind active throughout life can help maintain cognitive function and reduce the risk of dementia. Engage in activities that challenge your mind, such as learning a new language, playing brain-training games, or taking on new hobbies.

Taking Control of Your Aging Journey

By understanding the biological changes associated with aging and making informed lifestyle choices, you can significantly impact your health trajectory. Don't view aging as a passive process you have no control over. Embrace a proactive approach. Become an active participant in your own longevity. This book will equip you with the knowledge and tools to make informed decisions about your health and well-being, empowering you to live a long, healthy, and fulfilling life.

Remember, you are not defined by your age. You are defined by your choices and your zest for life. Let's embark on this journey together and unlock the incredible potential that lies within you for a vibrant and fulfilling future.

Chapter 2

Age is a Number, Not a Limitation - Dispelling Myths and Redefining Potential

Society often bombards us with negative stereotypes about aging. Images of frail figures and fading memories paint a bleak picture of our later years. But what if these stereotypes are nothing more than myths?

This chapter shatters these myths and empowers you to redefine what it means to age. We'll explore the incredible potential that lies within you, regardless of the number on your birth certificate.

Mythbusters: Debunking Common Misconceptions about Aging

Here are some of the most pervasive myths about aging, and the truths that lie beneath:

- Myth 1: Aging means decline.

While some physical changes are inevitable, this doesn't equate to decline. With a healthy lifestyle, you can maintain physical function, cognitive ability, and overall well-being well into your later years.

- Myth 2: You can't learn new things when you're older. Our brains are incredibly adaptable. Neuroplasticity, the brain's ability to change and form new connections throughout life, allows you to learn new skills, languages, and information at any age.

- Myth 3: Senior years are a time for isolation.

Social connection is crucial at every stage of life, and even more so as we age. Strong social bonds can improve physical and mental health, reduce loneliness, and foster a sense of purpose.

- Myth 4: You can't have a fulfilling career past a certain age.

Many individuals find their most fulfilling work later in life. Experience and wisdom gained over the years can make you a valuable asset in your field, or you can choose to pursue a completely new passion project.

- Myth 5: Retirement means inactivity.

Retirement is an opportunity to explore new interests, travel the world, volunteer in your community, or even start your own business.

Real People, Real Stories: Celebrating the Achievements of Older Adults

Here are some inspiring examples of older adults defying stereotypes and achieving remarkable feats:

- Grandma Moses: Anna Mary Robertson Moses, known as Grandma Moses, began painting in her late 70s and achieved international recognition for her vibrant and captivating folk art.

- Fauja Singh: Nicknamed "The Flying Sikh," Fauja Singh became the oldest person to complete a marathon at the age of 100, shattering records and inspiring others to pursue their athletic dreams.

- David Hockney: This renowned British artist continues to create captivating works well into his 80s, proving that creativity knows no age limit.

- Harriett Tubman: This iconic figure for freedom fought tirelessly for the abolition of slavery well into her 90s, demonstrating the power of resilience and purpose.

These are just a few examples. Countless individuals are rewriting the narrative of aging by pursuing passions, achieving goals, and making significant contributions to society, regardless of their age. You too can be one of them!

Unleashing Your Potential: Redefining what it Means to Thrive in Your Later Years

So, how do you tap into your potential and create a vibrant and fulfilling future? Here are some key strategies:

- Identify Your Passions: What ignites your curiosity? What activities bring you joy? Reconnect with old passions or explore new ones.

- Set Goals and Challenges: Having goals keeps you motivated and engaged. Set SMART goals (Specific, Measurable, Achievable, Relevant, and

Time-bound) to give your aspirations a roadmap for success.

•   Embrace Lifelong Learning: Never stop learning and exploring! Take classes, join a book club, attend lectures, or simply pick up a new hobby that challenges your mind.

•   Stay Active: Physical activity is crucial for maintaining physical and mental health. Find activities you enjoy, whether it's walking, swimming, dancing, or joining a fitness class for seniors.

•   Nurture Your Social Connections: Social interaction fosters a sense of belonging and reduces loneliness. Connect with friends and family, join social groups, volunteer your time, or participate in community events.

•   Embrace New Technology: Technology can be a powerful tool for staying connected, learning new skills, and managing your health. Explore various technological resources, and don't be afraid to seek help from younger generations.

Age is truly just a number. It doesn't define your potential, your capabilities, or your zest for life.

By challenging stereotypes, embracing lifelong learning, and nurturing your passions, you can rewrite the narrative of aging and create a future that is brimming with purpose, joy, and fulfillment.

**Ready to embark on this exciting journey? Let's explore some additional ways to dismantle limiting beliefs and unlock your true potential

Reframing Your Mindset: Shifting from Limitations to Possibilities

Our thoughts and beliefs have a profound impact on our experiences. If we hold onto limiting beliefs about aging, we may unconsciously sabotage our potential. Here are some strategies to reframe your mindset and embrace the possibilities that lie ahead:

• Challenge Negative Self-Talk: We all have that inner critic whispering doubts in our ears. Learn to recognize these negative thoughts and challenge them with positive affirmations. Instead of "I'm too old to learn that," reframe it as "I'm excited to explore new challenges and keep my mind sharp."

- Focus on Your Strengths: Don't dwell on perceived limitations. Instead, identify your strengths and experiences. What are you good at? What wisdom can you share with others? Leverage these strengths to pursue your goals and make a positive impact.

- Embrace New Experiences: Step outside your comfort zone and try new things. Take a dance class, learn a new language, or travel to a destination you've always dreamed of. Embrace the novelty of new experiences and the opportunities for growth they present.

- Find Inspiration: Surround yourself with positive role models who are thriving in their later years. Read biographies of inspiring older adults, watch documentaries, or connect with mentors who can offer guidance and support.

- Celebrate Every Milestone: No accomplishment is too small. Acknowledge and celebrate your progress, no matter how big or small. This will keep you motivated and reinforce your belief in your capabilities.

Turning Setbacks into Stepping Stones: Embracing Resilience

Life throws curveballs. Setbacks and challenges are inevitable. The key is not to let them define you. Develop resilience, the ability to bounce back from adversity and emerge stronger. Here are some tips:

•   Maintain a Positive Attitude: A positive outlook doesn't mean ignoring problems. It means acknowledging them while focusing on potential solutions and maintaining hope for the future.

•   Practice Gratitude: Take time each day to appreciate the good things in your life, big or small. Gratitude fosters a sense of well-being and can help you weather difficult times.

•   Seek Support: Don't be afraid to ask for help when you need it. Lean on friends, family, therapists, or support groups for emotional and practical assistance.

•   Focus on What You Can Control: Life is full of uncertainties. Focus your energy on the things you can control, such as your attitude, actions, and choices.

•   Learn from Your Experiences: Every setback presents a learning opportunity. Reflect on what you can take away from the experience to better equip yourself for the future.

Building a Supportive Network: Empowering Yourself and Others

The journey of aging is enriched by connection. Surrounding yourself with a supportive network of family, friends, and like-minded individuals can make a significant difference in your well-being. Here's how to build and nurture your support network:

•   Invest in Existing Relationships: Strengthen bonds with family and close friends. Spend quality time together, share your experiences, and offer support in return.

•   Expand Your Social Circles: Step outside your comfort zone and explore new social opportunities. Join a club, volunteer your time, or participate in community events.

•   Seek Mentorship: Connect with individuals who inspire you and can offer guidance based on their experiences.

•   Offer Mentorship: Share your wisdom and experiences with younger generations. Mentoring can be a rewarding way to give back and foster connection.

•   Embrace Intergenerational Relationships: Building relationships with people of all ages can be enriching. Learn from younger generations and share your life experiences with them.

By creating a strong support network, you not only enrich your own life but also contribute to a more connected and supportive community for all ages.

Conclusion: Age is a Journey, Not a Destination

Aging is not a process to be feared but rather a remarkable journey of growth, self-discovery, and continued contribution. By challenging limiting beliefs, embracing lifelong learning, and nurturing positive relationships, you can create a future filled with purpose, joy, and fulfillment.

This book will serve as your guide on this journey, providing you with the knowledge, tools, and inspiration to unlock your full potential and thrive in your later years. Remember, you are not defined by your age. You are defined by your choices, your resilience, and your unwavering spirit. Embrace the adventure that lies ahead!

Chapter 3

Nourishing Your Body - A Guide to Healthy Eating for Longevity

As we set out on this journey of sound aging, one of the most amazing assets available to us is food. The food sources we pick fuel our bodies, impact our energy levels, and assume a pivotal part in keeping up with physical and mental capability over the course of life. This chapter digs into the study of good dieting for life span, furnishing you with a guide to support your body for ideal prosperity.

The Food-Body Association: Understanding What Nourishment Means for Aging

The Aging system is affected by different variables, and one of the most huge is ongoing irritation. Persistent second rate irritation, frequently energized by an unfortunate eating regimen, can harm cells and tissues, add to various age-related illnesses, and speed up mental degradation.

Then again, an eating regimen wealthy in specific supplements and cancer prevention agents can assist with relieving irritation, advance cell wellbeing, and backing mental capability. How it's done:

•   Cancer prevention agents: These strong particles battle free revolutionaries, unsound atoms that harm cells and add to aggravation. Organic products, vegetables, and entire grains are amazing wellsprings of cancer prevention agents.

- Phytonutrients: These plant-based intensifies offer different medical advantages, including diminishing aggravation and shielding cells from harm. Cruciferous vegetables, berries, and vegetables are rich in phytonutrients.

- Omega-3 Unsaturated fats: These sound fats tracked down in greasy fish, pecans, and flaxseeds have been displayed to decrease aggravation, work on mental capability, and safeguard against coronary illness.

- Fiber: Fiber keeps you feeling full, controls glucose levels, and advances stomach wellbeing. A solid stomach microbiome is vital for general wellbeing and has been connected to a decreased gamble of constant illnesses.

Building a Plate for Life span: Fundamental Parts of a Sound Eating routine

All in all, what precisely would it be advisable for you to eat to advance sound aging? Here is a breakdown of the fundamental parts of a life span diet:

- Products of the soil: Go for the gold five servings of leafy foods everyday. Pick various varieties to boost your admission of various nutrients, minerals, and cancer prevention agents.

•   Entire Grains: Entire grains are a rich wellspring of fiber, complex starches, and fundamental nutrients. Settle on earthy colored rice, quinoa, entire wheat bread, and oats rather than refined grains.

•   Lean Protein: Protein is critical for keeping up with bulk and advancing satiety. Pick lean protein sources like fish, poultry, beans, vegetables, and nuts.

•   Solid Fats: While restricting soaked and undesirable fats, incorporate sound fats from sources like olive oil, avocado, nuts, and seeds in your eating routine. These fats give fundamental supplements and backing mental capability.

•   Low-Fat Dairy (Discretionary): Low-fat dairy items can be a decent wellspring of calcium and vitamin D, both significant for bone wellbeing. Nonetheless, a few people might have lactose narrow mindedness or pick a plant-based diet. Consult your primary care physician or an enrolled dietitian for customized direction.

•	Limit Added Sugars, Handled Food varieties, and Red Meat: Limit your admission of added sugars, refined carbs tracked down in handled food varieties, and red meat. These food sources can add to irritation and increment the gamble of constant illnesses.

Dietary Examples for Life span: Investigating Various Methodologies

There's nobody size-fits-all way to deal with smart dieting. The following are a couple of famous dietary examples that have been connected to life span:

•	The Mediterranean Eating regimen: This heart-sound eating routine stresses natural products, vegetables, entire grains, vegetables, fish, and solid fats from olive oil. Red meat and handled food varieties are devoured with some restraint.

•	The Scramble Diet: This dietary methodology centers around bringing down pulse and stresses natural products, vegetables, entire grains, low-fat dairy items, and lean protein. Red meat, salt, and added sugars are restricted.

•	The Brain Diet: Consolidating components of the Mediterranean and Run eats less, the Brain diet centers around mind wellbeing. It underscores verdant green vegetables, berries, nuts, entire grains, and fish while restricting red meat, immersed fats, and broiled food varieties.

•	The Plant-Based Diet: This diet focuses on organic products, vegetables, entire grains, vegetables, nuts, and seeds. Some plant-based diets might incorporate eggs and dairy items, while others are totally vegetarian.

Tracking down An ideal choice for You: Customizing Your Plate

The ideal eating regimen is one that is manageable, pleasant, and lines up with your singular requirements and inclinations. Here are a few methods for making a customized eating plan for life span:

•	Consider your medical issue and sensitivities: Consult your primary care physician or an enlisted dietitian to fit your eating regimen to address a particular wellbeing concerns you might have.

•   Investigate various cooking styles: Track down sound and heavenly recipes from different culinary customs to keep your dinners fascinating.

•   Cook more dinners at home: This permits you to control the fixings and part measures.

•   Peruse food names: Focus on serving sizes, immersed and unfortunate fat substance, added sugars, and sodium levels.

•   Careful eating: Dial back, relish your food, and focus on your body's craving and totality signs.

•   Remain hydrated: Drinking a lot of water over the course of the day is vital for general wellbeing and processing.

•   Be adaptable: Don't feel remorseful about periodic guilty pleasures. Center around settling on sound decisions more often than not.

Past the Plate: Extra Methodologies for Ideal Sustenance

A sound eating routine is only one piece of the riddle with regards to supporting your body for life span. Here are a few extra factors to consider:

•	Segment Control: Even good food varieties can add to weight gain whenever devoured in abundance. Practice segment control and utilize more modest plates to abstain from gorging.

•	Supplements (Consult your Doctor): Certain enhancements, like vitamin D and omega-3 unsaturated fats, might be gainful for certain people. Notwithstanding, talk about any expected enhancements with your primary care physician to guarantee they are protected and suitable for you.

•	Oversee Pressure: Ongoing pressure can disturb your craving and obstruct supplement retention. Practice stress management strategies like reflection, yoga, or profound breathing to advance unwinding and smart dieting propensities.

•	Keep a Solid Stomach Microbiome: The stomach microbiome assumes a pivotal part in processing, resistant capability, and general wellbeing. Support a sound stomach by devouring prebiotics (tracked down in natural products, vegetables, and entire grains) and probiotics (found in matured food sources like yogurt and kefir).

• 	Normal Dental Consideration: Keeping up with great oral cleanliness is fundamental for general wellbeing and could affect your eating regimen. Unfortunate dental wellbeing can make biting troublesome, prompting a restricted dietary admission.

To Embrace a Way of life of Sustenance

Supporting your body for life span isn't just about the food you eat. About making a sound way of life upholds your wellbeing. By joining a reasonable eating routine with other solid propensities, you can enable your body to flourish all through your journey.

Keep in mind, food isn't simply food; it's a useful asset for advancing wellbeing, forestalling sickness, and carrying on with a long and dynamic life. Investigate new flavors, try different things with sound recipes, and embrace a careful way to deal with eating. By sustaining your body, you are supporting your true capacity for a satisfying future.

Chapter 4

Moving Your Body - The Power of Exercise for Healthy Aging

As we age, remaining dynamic turns out to be significantly more critical for keeping up with physical and mental wellbeing. Practice isn't just about remaining in shape or looking great. It's an intense device for battling the impacts of aging, advancing life span, and upgrading your personal satisfaction.

This chapter jumps into the science behind practice for solid aging and gives viable techniques to integrating actual work into your day to day daily schedule, no matter what your ongoing wellness level.

The Study of Development: How Exercise Advantages Your Body and Brain

Practice gives a huge number of advantages to your body and brain as you age. How it's done:

- Actual Advantages:

o   Reduces Persistent Sickness Chance: Ordinary actual work oversees conditions like coronary illness, stroke, diabetes, a few sorts of disease, and hypertension.

o   Maintains Muscle Mass: Muscle loss is a characteristic piece of aging, yet work out, especially strength preparing, assists with muscling mass and further develop strength.

o   Improves Bone Thickness: Exercise, particularly weight-bearing exercises, keeps up with bone thickness and diminishes the gamble of osteoporosis.

o   Enhances Equilibrium and Coordination: Standard activity further develops equilibrium and coordination, diminishing the gamble of falls, a critical worry in more seasoned grown-ups.

o   Boosts Energy Levels: Active work battles weakness and increments energy levels, upgrading your general wellbeing.

•   Mental Advantages:

o   Sharpens Mental Capability: Exercise has been displayed to work on mental capability, memory, and concentration. It can assist with forestalling mental deterioration and diminish the gamble of dementia.

o   Elevates State of mind: Exercise advances the arrival of endorphins, chemicals that have temperament supporting impacts and can battle side effects of sadness and uneasiness.

o   Improves Rest Quality: Customary actual work can add to all the more likely rest quality, fundamental for generally speaking physical and emotional well-being.

o   Reduces Stress: Exercise can be an integral asset for overseeing pressure, advancing unwinding and mental wellbeing.

Viewing as Your Fit: Picking Activities You Appreciate

The way to staying with a work-out routine is finding exercises you really appreciate. There's nobody size-fits-all methodology. Here are a few choices to consider:

•   Cardio: Go for the gold 150 minutes of moderate-power oxygen consuming movement, like energetic strolling, cycling, swimming, or moving, most days of the week.

- Strength Preparing: Consolidate strength preparing practices something like two times per week to construct bulk and work on bone thickness. Bodyweight works out, free loads, or opposition groups are successful choices.

- Low-Effect Exercises: In the event that you have restrictions or wounds, low-influence practices like water heart stimulating exercise, yoga, or Pilates can give fantastic advantages.

- Equilibrium and Coordination Activities: Activities that challenge your equilibrium and coordination, for example, Judo or explicit yoga presents, can further develop fall anticipation.

- Bunch Wellness Classes: Joining a gathering wellness class can give social collaboration, inspiration, and a feeling of local area.

- Finding Exercises You Appreciate: Perhaps it's climbing, planting, hitting the dance floor with an accomplice, or playing sports. Pick exercises you view as tomfoolery and locking in.

Beginning Gradually and Continuously Advancing: Building a Manageable Everyday practice

Beginning another work-out routine can dismay. Here are a few hints to guarantee a protected and economical methodology:

•	Consult Your Doctor: Prior to beginning any new activity program, consult your doctor to talk about your wellbeing and get customized suggestions. This is especially significant assuming you have any current ailments.

•	Start Gradually: Begin with brief spans and slowly increase the recurrence and force of your exercises as your wellness level moves along.

•	Stand by listening to Your Body: Focus on your body's signs. Take rest days when required, and don't drive yourself to the mark of agony.

•	Put forth Practical Objectives: Put forth feasible objectives and keep tabs on your development. Celebrating little triumphs will keep you roused.

•	Track down an Exercise Mate: Having somebody to practice with can offer help, responsibility, and make your exercises more pleasant.

Beating Difficulties and Remaining Inspired

Staying with an activity program can challenge. Here are a few systems to defeat impediments and remain propelled:

•	Plan Your Exercises: Deal with practice like some other significant arrangement in your schedule.

•	Figure out an Opportunity that Works for You: Whether it's morning, evening, or night, pick a period that accommodates your timetable and energy levels.

•	Stir Up Your Daily schedule: To stay away from fatigue, attempt various activities and exercises to keep things fascinating.

•	Reward Yourself: Commend your accomplishments and achievements with non-food rewards.

•	Center around the Advantages: Remind yourself how great activity causes you to feel and the

positive effect it has on your wellbeing and prosperity.

•	Track down an Activity People group: Join a wellness class, strolling bunch, or online local community for help and inspiration.

•	Keep tabs on Your Development: Utilize a wellness tracker or diary to screen your advancement and praise your accomplishments.

•	Center around How You Feel: Don't simply zero in on weight reduction or style. Focus on how exercise further develops your energy levels, mind-set, and general wellbeing.

Practice Past the Exercise center Walls: Integrating Development Over the course of Your Day

Formal work-out schedules are essential, yet you can likewise consolidate development over the course of your day to build your general movement level. Here are a few thoughts:

•	Use the Staircase: Pick the steps at whatever point conceivable rather than the lift.

•	Park Further Away: Challenge yourself to stop further away from your destination and walk somewhat more.

•	Do Family Errands: Exercises like planting, yard work, or cleaning your home can give a moderate exercise.

•	Take Action Breaks: Get up and move around like clockwork to stay away from delayed sitting. Do some stretches, stroll around the workplace, or use the staircase a couple of times.

•	Integrate Active work into Your Side interests: Perhaps you appreciate moving, playing a game with companions, or taking a functioning get-away. Track down ways of incorporating development into your relaxation exercises.

Practice is a Festival of Your Body:

Keep in mind, practice isn't about discipline or accomplishing a specific constitution. It's a festival of your body's mind boggling potential. By integrating actual work into your life, you are putting resources into your wellbeing, prosperity, and eventually, your life span. Find exercises you appreciate, pay attention to your body, and steadily fabricate a manageable schedule that enables you to move with certainty and strength all through your later years.

Embrace the delight of development, and watch your body and psyche thrive!

Chapter 5

Sleep: The Foundation of Restoration - Habits for Deep and Rejuvenating Sleep for Healthy Aging

As we age, the significance of a decent night's rest turns out to be significantly more essential. Rest isn't just about feeling rested; it's the establishment for physical and mental wellbeing all through our lives. During rest, our bodies fix tissues, solidify recollections, and direct chemicals fundamental for by and large wellbeing. In any case, rest examples can change with age, making it more testing to accomplish the profound, supportive rest we hunger for.

This part plunges into the science behind rest and solid aging. We'll investigate the advantages of value rest, normal rest unsettling influences in more established grown-ups, and down to earth systems to develop a rest schedule that advances a tranquil evening and a better you.

The Advantages of Value Rest for healthy Aging

•   Worked on Mental Capability: Profound rest assumes an imperative part in memory union and learning. Satisfactory rest can upgrade concentration, fixation, and critical thinking skills.

•   Improved Actual Wellbeing: Rest is fundamental for cell fix and recovery. It fortifies the safe framework, manages chemicals that control hunger and digestion, and keeps a sound weight.

•   Reduced Risk of Chronic Disease: Lack of rest is connected to an expanded gamble of persistent medical conditions like coronary illness, stroke, diabetes, and, surprisingly, Alzheimer's sickness.

•   Boosted Emotional Wellbeing: Sufficient rest boost emotional wellbeing, lessens pressure and tension, and further develops mind-set.

Common Sleep Disturbances in Older Adults

•   Changes in Sleep Architecture: As we age, the amount of sleep normally diminishes, while lighter rest stages become more prominent. This can prompt divided sleep and frequent awakenings during the night.

•   Insomnia: Trouble nodding off or staying unconscious is a typical complain among older adults.

•   Rest Apnea: This condition makes breathing pause and begin over and over during rest, prompting unfortunate rest quality and daytime weakness.

•   Restless Legs Syndrome (RLS): This neurological issue causes an irresistible urge to move the legs, frequently at night, disrupting sleep.

•   Nocturia: The incessant need to pee during the night can essentially upset rest designs.

Developing a Rest Well disposed Daily schedule

Here are a pragmatic systems you can carry out to further develop your rest quality:

•   Lay out an Ordinary Rest Timetable: Hit the hay and wake up simultaneously every day, even on ends of the week, to control your body's normal rest wake cycle (circadian musicality).

•   Make a Loosening up Sleep time Schedule: Wind down before bed with quieting exercises like perusing, washing up, or paying attention to calming music. Abstain from invigorating exercises like sitting in front of the TV or involving electronic gadgets for essentially an hour prior to rest.

•   Streamline Your Rest Climate: Guarantee your room is dull, tranquil, cool, and mess free. Put resources into power outage shades, earplugs, and an agreeable sleeping pad and cushions.

•   Foster a Loosening up Pre-Rest Custom: Clean up, practice delicate yoga or contemplation, or read a quieting book before bed.

•   Limit Caffeine and Liquor Admission: Caffeine can slow down rest, particularly whenever consumed later in the day. While liquor might cause you to feel sluggish at first, it disturbs rest quality later in the evening.

- Standard Activity: Actual work advances better rest, yet stay away from demanding activity excessively near sleep time.

- Light Openness: Get standard openness to normal daylight during the day. This manages your circadian musicality and advances better rest around evening time.

- Oversee Pressure: Persistent pressure can altogether influence rest. Practice unwinding strategies like profound breathing, reflection, or yoga to oversee feelings of anxiety.

- See a Specialist if necessary: On the off chance that you experience determined rest issues, consult your doctor to preclude any fundamental ailments and examine treatment choices.

Extra Tips for Older Adults

- Limit Rests: Extended rests during the day can make it harder to nod off around evening time. Assuming that you do rest, keep it short (20-30 minutes) and try not to rest late in the early evening.

•	Be Aware of Night Dinners: Keep away from weighty feasts or fiery food varieties near sleep time, as they can cause stomach related distress and upset rest.

•	Remain Hydrated: Drying out can add to rest issues. Drink a lot of water over the course of the day, however keep away from unreasonable liquids just before sleep time.

•	Think about Light Treatment: In the event that you experience side effects of occasional emotional issue (Miserable), which can upset rest designs, light treatment might be valuable. Consult your doctor for direction.

By integrating these techniques into your daily schedule, you can further develop your rest quality and experience the various advantages of a decent night's rest. Keep in mind, sound rest propensities are an interest in your general wellbeing and prosperity, permitting you to carry on with a more dynamic and satisfying life as you age.

Chapter 6

Sharpen Your Mind: Brain Training and Activities to Enhance Cognitive Function for Healthy Aging

Our minds are momentous organs, with the possibility to remain sharp and versatile all through our lives. Very much like our bodies, our minds benefit from ordinary activity to keep up with ideal capability. This section dives into the universe of brain training and investigates different exercises intended to challenge your mental abilities, help memory, and upgrade mental capability as you age.

Why Brain Training Matters

• Worked on Mental Execution: Participating in brain training exercises can help keep up with or even further develop memory, handling speed, critical thinking abilities, and decisive abilities to reason.

• Improved Brain adaptability: The brain has a striking skill to adjust and shape new brain associations over the course of life, an interaction called brain adaptability. Mind training exercises can animate brain adaptability, keeping your brain nimble and responsive.

•	Decreased Hazard of Mental deterioration: Consistently testing your brain might assist deferral or even with forestalling age-related mental degradation and conditions like dementia.

•	More honed Psyche, More honed Life: Mind training exercises can improve concentration, focus, and general mental clarity, prompting a really satisfying and connection with life.

Mind Training Exercises: Fun and Successful Choices

•	Exemplary Games and Riddles: Crosswords, Sudoku, jigsaw riddles, and word look are immortal puzzles that challenge memory, jargon, and critical thinking abilities.

•	Mastering Another Expertise: Whether it's another dialect, an instrument, or an imaginative pursuit like canvas or photography, gaining some new useful knowledge invigorates mental capability and keeps your brain locked in.

•	Mind Training Applications and Web based Games: Various applications and internet games offer brain training practices that target explicit mental abilities like memory, consideration, and handling speed.

•	Tabletop games and Games: Messing around like chess, Scrabble, or extension with companions or family gives a social component while testing your mental abilities in a tomfoolery and intelligent way.

•	Perusing and Composing: Perusing animates your brain by presenting you to new data and thoughts, while composing connects with memory, jargon, and decisive reasoning abilities.

•	Care and Contemplation: These practices advance concentration, fixation, and present-second mindfulness, which can work on mental capability and by and large wellbeing.

•	Actual work: Customary activity isn't only really great for your body; it's useful for your brain as well. Active work increases blood stream to the brain, advancing brain adaptability and mental capability.

Tips for Viable Mind Training

•	Assortment is Vital: Don't become trapped in a hopeless cycle! Pick an assortment of mind training exercises to challenge different mental spaces and keep your exercises intriguing.

•	Begin Little and Continuously Increase Effort Start with practices that are testing yet attainable, and bit by bit increase your effort as your abilities move along.

•	Regularly practice it: Consistency is vital. Mean to take part in brain training exercises for no less than 20-30 minutes most days of the week.

•	Center around the Journey: Mind training is a deep rooted venture, not a rush to the end goal. Partake during the time spent learning and testing yourself.

•	Mingle and Associate: Participating in brain training exercises with companions or family can add a social component and make the cycle more charming.

Past Mind Training: Way of life Propensities for Mental Wellbeing

•	Sound Eating routine: An eating regimen wealthy in organic products, vegetables, entire grains, and lean protein gives your brain the supplements it requires to ideally work.

•	Quality Rest: Satisfactory rest is fundamental for mental capability. Hold back nothing long periods of rest every evening.

•	Oversee Pressure: Persistent pressure can adversely affect mental capability. Practice unwinding procedures like profound breathing, reflection, or yoga to oversee feelings of anxiety.

•	Remain Hydrated: Parchedness can prompt weakness and hindered mental capability. Drink a lot of water over the course of the day.

By consolidating mind training exercises and embracing solid way of life propensities, you can enable your brain to remain sharp, drew in, and strong all through your brilliant years. Keep in mind, a solid brain is a blissful mind, permitting you to encounter the delights of long lasting learning and a functioning, satisfying life.

Chapter 7

Building a Strong Partnership: Your Doctor - The Key to Healthy Aging

Regular checkups and preventive measures are essential for healthy aging. However, a strong relationship with your doctor goes beyond simply scheduling appointments. It's about building trust, open communication, and a collaborative approach to managing your health. This chapter explores the importance of a positive doctor-patient relationship and equips you with tips for effective communication and maximizing the benefits of your preventive healthcare visits.

Why a Strong Doctor-Patient Relationship Matters

•   Improved Health Outcomes: Open communication allows your doctor to understand your unique health concerns and preferences, leading to more personalized and effective care plans.

•   Early Detection of Health Issues: A doctor familiar with your medical history can identify potential problems early on, when they are often easier to treat.

•   Enhanced Preventive Care: Your doctor can tailor preventive measures like screenings and vaccinations to your specific needs and risk factors.

- Increased Confidence and Trust: Knowing you have a reliable healthcare partner can provide peace of mind and empower you to take charge of your health.

Building a Strong Foundation: Communication is Key

- Be Prepared: Come to appointments with a list of questions and concerns.

- Be Clear and Concise: Explain your symptoms and medical history in detail.

- Ask Questions: Don't hesitate to ask for clarification or seek additional information.

- Be Open and Honest: Discuss your lifestyle habits, including diet, exercise, and any medications you take.

- Express Your Preferences: Let your doctor know your preferred communication style and any concerns you have regarding treatment options.

Making the Most of Your Doctor's Visits

- Schedule Regular Checkups: The frequency of your visits will depend on your age, overall health, and risk factors. Discuss a checkup schedule with your doctor.

•	Arrive Early: This allows time to complete paperwork and reduces stress before your appointment.

•	Bring Relevant Medical Records: If you're switching doctors or have recent test results, bring copies for your new doctor.

•	Take Notes: Jot down key points discussed during your appointment and any follow-up instructions.

•	Don't Be Afraid to Seek Second Opinions: If you're unsure about a diagnosis or treatment plan, discuss the possibility of seeking a second opinion with your doctor.

Preventive Measures for Healthy Aging

•	Annual Checkups: These visits allow your doctor to monitor your overall health, discuss any concerns you may have, and recommend preventive screenings.

•	Preventive Screenings: Regular screenings can detect potential health problems like cancer, heart disease, and diabetes in their early stages, leading to more effective treatment. Common screenings for older adults include blood pressure checks, cholesterol tests, mammograms, colonoscopies, and bone density scans.

•	Vaccinations: Stay up-to-date on vaccinations like the flu shot and shingles vaccine, which can help prevent serious illnesses.

•	Develop a Healthy Lifestyle: Partner with your doctor to create a personalized plan for a healthy diet, regular exercise, and adequate sleep.

Remember: You are an active participant in your healthcare journey. By building a strong relationship with your doctor, advocating for your needs, and taking a proactive approach to preventive care, you can empower yourself to achieve a healthy and fulfilling life as you age.

Chapter 8

Common Age-Related Conditions: Understanding Risk Factors and Early Detection Strategies for Healthy Aging

As we age, our bodies normally change. While these progressions are a typical piece of life, they can likewise increase our risk of fostering specific medical issues. This part investigates the absolute most normal age-related conditions, enabling you to comprehend your risk factors, distinguish early warning signs, and investigate techniques for early location. By being proactive about your wellbeing, you can assume an essential part in dealing with these circumstances and keeping up with your wellbeing all through your brilliant years.

Understanding Risk Variables

A few elements can impact your risk of creating age-related conditions. Here are a few key contemplations:

•   Age: Sequential age is a critical risk factor for some age-related conditions.

•   Family Ancestry: Having a family background of specific circumstances, like coronary illness, diabetes, or Alzheimer's sickness, can increase your risk.

•	Way of life Propensities: Diet, exercise, smoking, and liquor utilization all assume a part in your wellbeing and can fundamentally affect your risk for different circumstances.

•	Weight: Conveying abundance weight can expand your risk for coronary illness, diabetes, and certain diseases.

Normal Age-Related Conditions and Early Location Systems

1. Heart Disease

•	Risk Variables: Hypertension, elevated cholesterol, diabetes, smoking, family ancestry.

•	Early Location: Ordinary tests to screen circulatory strain and cholesterol levels.

•	Techniques: Solid eating routine, customary activity, smoking end, overseeing pressure.

2. Stroke

•	Risk Variables: Hypertension, elevated cholesterol, diabetes, smoking, atrial fibrillation (unpredictable heartbeat).

- Early Identification: Ordinary tests to screen pulse and cholesterol levels.

- Systems: Same as coronary illness, in addition to overseeing atrial fibrillation if present.

3. Cancer

- Risk Elements: Age, family ancestry, way of life factors like smoking and sun openness, certain hereditary changes.

- Early Recognition: Normal screenings suggested by your doctor, like mammograms, colonoscopies, and prostate tests (for men).

- Methodologies: Solid eating regimen, keeping a sound weight, sun insurance, immunizations like HPV antibody (for specific age gatherings).

4. Diabetes

- Risk Elements: Family ancestry, stoutness, actual idleness, certain identities.

- Early Recognition: Glucose tests during customary exams.

- Techniques: Solid eating routine, customary activity, weight the executives, meds as endorsed by your doctor.

5. Arthritis

• Risk Elements: Age, family ancestry, past wounds, corpulence.

• Early Recognition: Agony, solidness, and enlarging in joints. Consult your doctor assuming side effects continue.

• Methodologies: Keeping a solid weight, exercise to keep up with joint portability, non-intrusive treatment, pain management techniques.

6. Osteoporosis

• Risk Variables: Age, female sex, family ancestry, low bone thickness, hormonal changes (menopause in ladies).

• Early Location: Bone thickness examines (DXA checks) as suggested by your primary care physician.

• Methodologies: Calcium and vitamin D rich eating routine, weight-bearing activities, meds as endorsed by your primary care physician.

7. Dementia (including Alzheimer's Illness)

• Risk Variables: Age, family ancestry, head wounds, certain way of life factors.

- Early Recognition: Cognitive decline, trouble concentrating, changes in conduct or character. Consult your primary care physician assuming you notice any disturbing changes.

- Methodologies: Intellectually invigorating exercises, remaining socially connected with, sound eating routine, great rest cleanliness, overseeing basic medical issue.

8. Vision and Hearing Loss

- Risk Variables: Age, family ancestry, openness to uproarious clamors (hearing loss).

- Early Discovery: Ordinary eye tests and hearing tests as suggested by your doctor.

- Systems: Shielding your eyes from UV beams with shades, utilizing portable hearing assistants if essential, keeping a sound eating routine.

Keep in mind: Early Recognition is Vital

By understanding your risk factors and the early warning indications of normal age-related conditions, you can make proactive strides towards early identification and the management. Standard wellbeing examinations, preventive screenings, and a sound way of life are the foundations of healthy aging.. Feel free to discuss any worries you might have with your doctor. By cooperating, you can make a customized plan to improve your wellbeing and prosperity as you age.

Chapter 9

Preventive Screenings and Tests: A Guide to Staying Ahead of Potential Health Issues for Healthy Aging

Preventive screenings and tests assume an essential part in proactive medical care for more older adults. These methodology can identify potential medical conditions from the get-go, when they are frequently more straightforward to treat and make due. This section furnishes you with a far reaching manual for normal preventive screenings and tests suggested for healthy aging.

Why Preventive Screenings Matter

•   Early Location: Numerous illnesses, like cancer, heart disease, and diabetes, can be effectively treated when trapped in their beginning phases. Preventive screenings can distinguish these circumstances before they cause huge side effects.

•   Further developed Treatment Results: Early intercession frequently prompts better treatment results and a greater of life.

•   Genuine serenity: Normal screenings can give inward feeling of harmony by identifying expected issues or affirming great wellbeing.

Who Chooses When to Get Screened?

The choice of when and how frequently to get screened relies upon a few elements, including:

•   Your Age: Screening suggestions differ in light age and chance elements.

•	Your Wellbeing History: Certain ailments or a family background of a particular illness might warrant more successive screenings.

•	Your General Wellbeing: Your primary care physician will consider your general wellbeing and chance elements to suggest fitting screenings.

Examining preventive screenings with your primary care physician at your ordinary checkups is pivotal. They can tailor a customized screening plan in light of your singular requirements.

Normal Preventive Screenings and Tests for More seasoned Grown-ups

Kind of Screening, What it Detects, Who Ought to Get Screened And Frequency

Circulatory strain Check

It detects High blood pressure. All adults need to get screened annually at least.

Cholesterol Test

It detects High cholesterol. Adults matured 40-75 (more continuous if high risk) are to get screened every 5 years (more regular if high gamble)

Glucose Test

It detects Diabetes. Adults with risk factors are to get screened every 3 years (more successive if high gamble)

Colonoscopy

It detects Colorectal cancer.

Adults matured 45-75 (sooner if high risk) are to get screened every 10 years (different choices accessible)

Mammography

It detects Breast cancer.

Women matured 50-74 (prior or later in light of risk) are to get screened every 1-2 years (different choices accessible)

Pap Smear Test

It detects Cervical cancer.

Women matured 21-65 (less successive after specific models met) are to get screened every 3-5 years (co-testing with HPV test conceivable)

Bone Thickness Scan

It detects Osteoporosis. Women matured 65+ and men matured 50+ with not set in stone by your doctor.

Extra Screenings:

•	Skin Malignant growth Screening: Standard self-assessments and expert skin tests by a specialist are suggested for all grown-ups.

•	Hearing Test: Customary hearing tests are prescribed for more seasoned grown-ups to distinguish hearing misfortune.

•	Vision Test: Complete eye tests are suggested each 1-2 years for grown-ups.

•	Dental Tests: Standard dental exams and cleanings are fundamental for keeping up with great oral wellbeing.

Keep in mind: Information is Power

Being educated about preventive screenings and tests enables you to assume responsibility for your wellbeing. Examine your singular requirements and hazard factors with your primary care physician to make a customized screening plan. Early identification is basic for fruitful treatment and a better you!

Chapter 10

The Fountain of Youth: How Strong Connections Lead to Healthy Aging

We as a whole know the significance of healthy habits like eating right and practicing for a long and satisfying life. However, there's one more impressive fixing in the recipe for healthy aging: solid social associations.

Research reliably shows that supporting cozy associations with family, companions, and community members significantly affects our wellbeing as we age. It's not just about feeling far better (however that is significant as well!). Social association can:

•	Boost Physical Health: Studies suggest strong social ties can bring down the risk of chronic diseases like heart disease and stroke. Social help may likewise empower solid ways of behaving like regular exercise and can promote a sense of accountability.

•	Hone your Brain: Social collaboration keeps your brain dynamic and connected with, which can assist with warding off mental degradation and dementia. Sharing encounters, learning new things together, and basically having discussions can all animate your mental muscles.

- Safeguard your psychological wellbeing: Dejection and segregation are significant risk factors for wretchedness and tension. Solid connections give a cradle against pressure, offer daily reassurance during difficult stretches, and provide you a feeling of having a place and motivation.

- Increase Life Expectancy: Research shows that socially associated individuals will quite often live longer than the people who are disengaged. The positive physical and psychological well-being benefits probably add to this life span.

Building Your Group of friends: It's Never too Late

Fortunately developing solid social connections is never too late. Here are a few hints to kick you off:

- Reconnect with lifelong companions and family: Contact individuals you haven't found in some time. A straightforward call, email, or greeting to espresso can revive old kinships.

•   Join a club or gathering: Find a gathering that shares your inclinations, whether it's a book club, a mobile gathering, or a worker association. This is an extraordinary method for meeting new individuals who appreciate comparative things.

•   Engage locally: Volunteer your chance to a neighborhood cause, go to community occasions, or take a class at a public venue.

•   Embrace innovation: Remain associated with friends and family who live far away through video calls, online entertainment (utilized carefully), or email.

•   Be an old buddy: Solid connections are a two-way road. Show up for your friends and family, offer help, and be a decent audience.

Keep in mind, areas of strength for building takes time and exertion. Show restraint, put yourself out there, and partake during the time spent supporting the connections that will advance your life all through your brilliant years.

Chapter 11
Finding Your Spark: Activities and Engagement for a Meaningful Life in Healthy Aging

As we age, our needs and viewpoints shift. What gave us pleasure in our more youthful years may never again hold a similar flash. Yet, the longing for reason and a satisfying life stays solid. The uplifting news is, healthy aging isn't just about actual wellbeing; about embracing additional opportunities and finding exercises light your energy. Here is your manual for starting happiness and reason in your brilliant years:

Rediscover Your Interests:

•	Ponder the Past: Go on an outing through a world of fond memories. What exercises did you appreciate in your more youthful years? Did you have side interests you put on pause because of work or family responsibilities? Maybe now is the ideal time to return to those failed to remember interests.

•	Investigate New Interests: Learn constantly! Take a class in something you've forever been interested about, such as painting, photography, or even another dialect. Investigate neighborhood studios or web based learning stages.

•	Embrace Imagination: Communicate your thoughts inventively through composition, music, dance, or in any event, cultivating. Innovative pursuits can be a strong wellspring of bliss and self-disclosure.

Exercises for Reason and Importance:

•	Volunteer Your Time: Reward your community and offer your abilities and experience. Chipping in can be unquestionably fulfilling, associating you with others and having a constructive outcome on the world.

•	Tutor Others: Offer your insight and involvement in more youthful ages. Propose to tutor a youthful expert, mentor a young games group, or volunteer at a nearby school.

•	Seek after Long lasting Learning: Challenge constantly yourself mentally. Take online courses, go to talks and studios, or join a book club.

•	Travel and Investigate: Experience new societies, expand your perspectives, and make enduring recollections. Consider joining travel bunches explicitly intended for older adults and seniors.

Taking part in Friendly Exercises:

•	Interface with Loved ones: Sustain your current connections and construct new ones. Plan standard trips with friends and family, join a social club, or take part in community occasions.

•	Embrace Innovation: Remain associated with friends and family who live far away through video calls, web-based entertainment (utilized carefully), or internet gaming networks for seniors.

•	Join a Wellness Class: Get dynamic and social simultaneously. There are wellness classes intended for all capacities, from delicate yoga to move classes. You'll work on your actual wellbeing and associate with other people who share your objectives.

Tracking down Reason in Day to day existence:

•	Center around Self-improvement: Challenge yourself to gain some new useful knowledge each day, whether it's another recipe, a verifiable reality, or another word. Connect with your brain and keep it sharp.

•	Practice Appreciation: Consider the positive parts of your life, enormous or little. Appreciation has been displayed to build satisfaction and wellbeing.

•	Embrace Care: Get some margin to dial back and value the current second. Practice contemplation, profound breathing activities, or just invest energy in nature.

•	Help other people: Even little thoughtful gestures can have a major effect. Propose to assist a neighbor, hold the entryway with opening for somebody, or essentially offer a grin.

Keep in mind: There's nobody size-fits-all way to deal with tracking down reason. The key is to investigate various exercises, embrace new encounters, and find what really lights your energy.

Extra Tips:

•	Make it a point to step outside your usual range of familiarity.

•	Begin little and step by step expand upon your exercises.

•	Center around the journey, in addition to the objective.

•	Find a responsibility accomplice to assist you with remaining propelled.

•	Above all, have a good time!

By taking part in exercises that give you pleasure and motivation, you'll improve your life as well as add to a better and seriously satisfying aging experience.

Chapter 12
Weathering the Storms: Strategies for Managing Stress and Cultivating Resilience for Healthy Aging

As we age, life definitely tosses curves. From wellbeing worries to changes in our day to day environments, stress can turn into a steady friend. However, here's the uplifting news: you can develop strength, the capacity to return from difficulties and keep up with profound wellbeing. Here are a few strong procedures to manage stress and construct strength for a more quiet and more joyful brilliant age:

Stress Management Procedures:

•   Recognize Your Stressors: The initial step is to comprehend what sets off your pressure. Is it monetary concerns, wellbeing concerns, or relationship issues? When you distinguish your stressors, you can foster methods for dealing with especially difficult times.

•   Practice Unwinding Strategies: Methods like profound breathing activities, reflection, and moderate muscle unwinding can assist with quieting your psyche and body notwithstanding pressure.

•   Challenge Negative Reasoning: Our considerations fundamentally impact our feelings of anxiety. Figure out how to recognize and challenge negative idea designs. Replace them with more sensible and positive self-talk.

•   Keep a Healthy Lifestyle: A fair eating regimen, customary activity, and satisfactory sleep are fundamental for managing stress and advancing in general wellbeing.

•   Limit Liquor and Caffeine: While these substances might appear to be loosening up temporarily, they can really deteriorate nervousness and sleep issues over the long haul.

Building Flexibility:

•	Foster an Uplifting perspective: Develop a hopeful demeanor. Center around the things you have some control over and track down the silver lining in tough spots.

•	Practice Appreciation: Finding opportunity to see the value in the beneficial things in your day to day existence, regardless of how little, can altogether help your mind-set and versatility.

•	Sustain Solid Connections: Solid social associations offer emotional help and a feeling of having a place, which are vital for versatility. Invest energy with friends and family, join a gathering, or volunteer locally.

•	Embrace a Development Outlook: View difficulties as any open doors for learning and development. This attitude encourages versatility and permits you to return from difficulties.

•	Center around Control: Engage yourself by zeroing in on the things you have some control over in your life. Figure out how to relinquish what you can't change and zero in on your responses and reactions.

•   Look for Proficient Assistance: Assuming pressure feels overpowering or you're battling to adapt, go ahead and seek for proficient assistance. A specialist can give significant instruments and methodologies to managing stress and working on profound wellbeing.

Extra Tips:

•   Practice care: Focus on the current second without judgment. This can assist with diminishing stress and increase sensations of quietness.

•   Participate in exercises you appreciate: Set aside a few minutes for side interests and exercises that give you pleasure and unwinding.

•   Associate with nature: Investing energy outside has been displayed to lessen pressure and further develop state of mind.

•   Figure out how to say no: Don't over-burden yourself. It's alright to define limits and decline demands that would add superfluous pressure to your life.

Keep in mind: Building versatility is a journey, not a destination. By integrating these methodologies into your day to day existence, you can foster the inward strength and survival strategies to explore life's difficulties and partake in a seriously satisfying and peaceful brilliant age.

Chapter 13
Securing Your Golden Years: A Guide to Financial Planning for Healthy Aging

Monetary security is a foundation of a tranquil and satisfying retirement. By preparing and settling on savvy monetary choices, you can guarantee your brilliant years are loaded up with autonomy, opportunity, and the capacity to seek after your interests. Here is a guide to explore your monetary journey for an effortless future:

Surveying What is happening:

• Assemble Your Archives: Begin by gathering all your monetary reports, including bank statements, speculation records, retirement account articulations, and any obligation records.

• Ascertain Your Pay and Costs: Track your month to month pay from all sources, including annuities, government managed retirement benefits, and any seasonal work pay. Compute your month to month expenses for basics like accommodation, food, utilities, and medical care. This will provide you with a reasonable image of your ongoing financial standing.

•	Gauge Your Retirement Needs: Think about your ideal retirement way of life. Will you travel widely? Scale back your day to day environment? Consider potential medical services costs and long haul care needs. This will assist you with deciding the amount you want to put something aside for retirement.

Building a Retirement Savings:

•	Maximize Employer supported retirement plans: If you have access to a 401(k) or comparable arrangement, contribute as much as your budget allows to take advantage of employer matching programs.

•	Put resources into Individual Retirement Records (IRAs): IRAs offer expense benefits for retirement investment funds. Customary IRAs offer duty deductible commitments with charge conceded development, while Roth IRAs offer tax-exempt withdrawals in retirement.

•	Investigate Other Speculation Choices: Consider expanding your portfolio with stocks, securities, and shared assets to oversee risk and augment returns. Counsel a monetary guide for customized proposals in light of your gamble resistance and time skyline.

•	Pay Off Debts: Exorbitant interest debts can essentially deplete your retirement reserve funds. Focus on taking care of MasterCards and other expensive loans to let loose your pay for saving.

Methodologies for Long haul Monetary Security:

•	Defer Retirement: If conceivable, consider working a couple of extra years past your underlying retirement age. This permits you to keep adding to your retirement reserve funds and amplify your Federal retirement aide benefits.

•	Scale back Your Day to day environment: Moving to a more modest home or loft can essentially diminish your lodging costs, opening up assets for different costs.

•	Investigate Federal medical insurance Choices: As you approach retirement age, really get to know Government medical care choices and supplemental protection intends to guarantee sufficient wellbeing inclusion.

•	Think about Long haul Care Protection: While not fundamental for everybody, long haul care protection can assist with taking care of the expenses of helped residing or nursing home consideration, safeguarding your retirement savings.

•	Make a Will and Legal authority: Domain arranging guarantees your resources are conveyed by your desires. A Legal authority permits somebody you trust to settle on monetary choices for your sake in the event that you can't do as such.

Extra Tips:

•	Foster a Financial plan and Track Your Spending: Make a reasonable financial plan and track your costs to recognize regions where you can scale back and save more.

•	Look for Proficient Assistance: A financial counselor can give customized direction in light of your monetary objectives and chance resistance.

•	Remain Informed: Teach yourself on monetary matters and stay up with the latest on changes in charge guidelines and retirement benefits.

•	Live Well Inside Your Means: While partaking in your brilliant years, be aware of your ways of managing money. Abstain from overspending and focus on long haul monetary security.

Keep in mind: Monetary making arrangements for retirement is a continuous cycle. Routinely survey your monetary methodology, change your arrangements on a case by case basis, and adjust to evolving conditions. By assuming responsibility for your funds today, you can fabricate a protected starting point for a blissful, sound, and free future.

Chapter 14

Aging in Place with Comfort and Confidence: Creating a Safe and Supportive Home

As we age, the craving to stay autonomous and live serenely in our own homes frequently develops further. Fortunately, with a couple of key changes, your home can be changed into a protected and strong shelter for ideal aging set up. Here is an extensive manual for establishing a climate that cultivates freedom, limits fall dangers, and upgrades your general wellbeing:

Evaluating Your Requirements:

•   Begin with a Security Stroll Through: Go for a sluggish stroll through your home, envisioning yourself utilizing regular things and exploring various spaces. Recognize regions that could present difficulties, like elusive floors, unfortunate lighting, or tight moving spaces.

•   Think about Future Necessities: While arranging adjustments, calculate expected changes in your portability or vision. Future-proofing your home can save you cash and hassles down the line.

•   Include Family and Experts: Examine your aging set up objectives with relatives and consider consulting a specialist for a customized evaluation and change proposals.

Key Changes for Security and Openness:

•   Restroom Security: This is a high-risk zone for falls. Introduce snatch bars close to the latrine, bath/shower, and by the sink. Think about a stroll in shower with an implicit seat and a handheld showerhead. Pick non-slip mats inside and outside the shower/tub.

•   Kitchen Security: Guarantee legitimate lighting over ledges and burners. Replace cabinet door handles with more straightforward to-hold handles. Lower every now and again utilized racks for better availability. Introduce switch dealt with fixtures for simpler activity. Consider adding differentiating hued tape to bureau edges to further develop perceivability.

•   Further developed Lighting: Introduce more splendid lighting all through the house, particularly in lobbies, flights of stairs, and entrances. Consider nightlights in the room and restroom for evening time route. Use movement sensor lights in habitually involved regions for added accommodation.

•   Flooring: Swap free carpets and select non-slip flooring materials like overlay, vinyl, or finished tiles. Guarantee appropriate covering with low heap and secure edges.

•   Flight of stairs Security: Introduce strong handrails on the two sides of flights of stairs. Consider adding differentiating shaded tape to the main edge of every step move toward further develop perceivability. Investigate the chance of introducing a stairlift in the event that steps become a huge test.

•   Entryways: Enlarge entryways if important to handily oblige wheelchairs or walkers more. Replace door handles with switch handles for simpler opening and shutting.

Extra Contemplations for Solace and Freedom:

•   General Plan Standards: Consolidate all inclusive plan standards whenever the situation allows. This implies making a space that is usable by individuals, everything being equal, paying little heed to mature or actual constraints.

•	Savvy Home Innovation: Investigate shrewd home gadgets like voice-initiated lighting controls, indoor regulators, and apparatuses to improve accommodation and autonomy.

•	Seating with Great Back Help: Put resources into agreeable seats with great back and arm backing to advance appropriate stance and lessen strain.

•	Clear Pathways: Guarantee clear and cleaned up pathways all through the house to limit stumbling risks.

•	Crisis Ready Frameworks: Think about introducing a clinical ready framework for added genuine serenity, permitting you to call for help if there should be an occurrence of a crisis.

Keep in mind: Aging set up is a journey, and your necessities might develop over the long haul. Consistently survey your home climate and make changes on a case by case basis. Make it a point to seek help from family, companions, or experts to guarantee your home keeps on being a protected and steady sanctuary for a satisfying and free life.

Chapter 15
Navigating Your Senior Living Options: A Guide to Assisted Living Communities and Beyond

As we age, our requirements and inclinations for everyday environments can change. While certain seniors value their freedom and expect to progress in years set up, others might need extra help to keep up with their personal satisfaction. This guide investigates senior living choices, including helped living networks, to assist you with settling on informed choices for a satisfying and secure future.

Grasping Your Requirements:

•   Freedom versus Support: Assess your ongoing degree of freedom and the level of help you might require with day to day exercises like washing, dressing, drug management, or housekeeping.

•   Socialization versus Protection: Think about your social inclinations. Do you flourish in common settings or lean toward a more confidential climate?

•	Monetary Contemplations: Research the expenses related with various senior living choices and calculate your spending plan and long haul monetary plans.

•	Area and Conveniences: Contemplate your ideal area. Would you like to remain nearby loved ones or would you say you are available to new environmental factors? Consider the significance of conveniences like nearby medical care, wellness offices, or transportation administrations.

Senior Living Choices: A Range of Care:

1. **Autonomous Living People group:**

•	Ideal for dynamic seniors who esteem their autonomy however want a social and upkeep free way of life.

•	Offer confidential condos or cabins with conveniences like housekeeping, eating corridors, and social exercises.

•	Inhabitants are regularly answerable for their own day to day living exercises.

2. Helped Living People group:

•   Give a strong climate to seniors who need some help with day to day exercises of living (ADLs) like washing, dressing, or drug management.

•   Offer private or semi-private lofts with housekeeping, dinners, and individual consideration administrations.

•   May have nearby medical services experts and deal social exercises and conveniences.

3. Proceeding with Care Retirement People group (CCRCs):

•   Offer a full continuum of care, from free living to helped living and talented nursing care, all on one grounds.

•   Furnish inhabitants with the adaptability to progress to more elevated levels of care as their necessities change.

•   Ordinarily require an extra charge and month to month administration expenses.

4. In-Home Consideration:

- • Permits seniors to stay in their own homes while getting help with everyday exercises.

- • Administrations can go from friendship and housekeeping to individual consideration and talented nursing care.

- • Offers a serious level of personalization and freedom.

5. 55+ Dynamic Grown-up Networks:

- • Age-confined networks intended for dynamic and free seniors.

- • Offer confidential homes or townhouses with conveniences like social clubs, wellness focuses, and sporting offices.

- • Inhabitants are ordinarily answerable for their own everyday living exercises.

Picking the Ideal Choice:

- • Think about your current and future requirements.

- • Include your family in conversations.

- • Visit different senior living networks and clarify some pressing issues.

•	Figure your financial plan and long haul monetary plans.

•	Make sure to look for proficient direction from a senior consideration guide.

Extra Contemplations:

•	Free living networks can be an extraordinary choice for seniors who are still generally autonomous yet partake in the social parts of a community setting.

•	Helped living networks give a steady climate to the individuals who need some assistance with everyday exercises.

•	CCRCs offer true serenity realizing that care choices are accessible on location if necessary later on.

•	In-home consideration permits seniors to stay in their recognizable environmental elements while getting the help they need.

•	55+ Dynamic Grown-up Networks take care of dynamic seniors who need a social and convenience rich living climate.

Keep in mind: There's no one size-fits-all answer for senior living. The most ideal choice for you will rely upon your singular necessities, inclinations, and financial plan. Through cautiously thinking about your choices and including your friends and family in the dynamic cycle, you can pick a senior living game plan that cultivates your wellbeing, freedom, and by and large personal satisfaction.

Chapter 16

Bridging the Gap: Technology Tools and Resources to Enhance Daily Activities for a Connected Life

Innovation is as of now not only for the youthful. Today, a huge swath of easy to use instruments and assets can engage seniors to remain associated, deal with their wellbeing, and work on regular errands. Here is a brief look into the tech tool stash that can upgrade your day to day existence and keep you associated:

Communication and Social Association:

•	Video Calling Applications: Remain associated with friends and family who live far away through video calls utilizing applications like WhatsApp, Facebook, Skype, or Zoom. See their countenances, share stories, and appreciate virtual visits from the solace of your home.

•	Online Entertainment Platforms: Platforms like Facebook or Nextdoor can assist you with associating with companions, family, and, surprisingly, nearby networks with comparable interests. Join gatherings, share updates, and remain in the know about nearby occasions.

•	Informing Applications: Informing applications like WhatsApp or Courier offer a relaxed and helpful method for keeping in contact with friends and family over the course of the day. Send fast messages, share photographs, and appreciate moment correspondence.

Wellbeing and Health Management:

•	Wellness Trackers and Smartwatches: These wearable gadgets track your means, pulse, sleep examples, and, surprisingly, offer delicate suggestions to remain dynamic. Screen your wellbeing information and remain inspired on your wellness process.

•	Telehealth Applications: Interface with specialists practically through telehealth applications. Plan arrangements, get conferences, and deal with your wellbeing worries from the solace of your home.

•	Medicine Management Applications: At absolutely no point ever miss a portion in the future! Medicine management applications assist you with setting updates, track meds, and even reorder remedies electronically.

Day to day existence Rearrangements:

•	Brilliant Home Gadgets: Improve on ordinary undertakings with savvy home gadgets. Control lights, indoor regulators, and machines with your voice or cell phone. Envision turning on the lights before you even get up or changing the room temperature from a distance.

•	Online Shopping for food and Conveyance: Get your regular food items conveyed directly to your doorstep! Peruse online stores, add things to your truck, and timetable a helpful conveyance time. Not any more weighty sacks to convey!

•	Ride-Sharing Applications: Need a ride? Ride-sharing applications like Uber or Lyft interface you with drivers at the tap of a button. Appreciate advantageous and reasonable transportation at whatever point you really want it.

Learning and Amusement:

•	Internet Learning Platforms: Learn constantly! Platforms like Coursera or edX offer a huge range of online seminars on for all intents and purposes any theme you can envision. Grow your insight, investigate new interests, and challenge yourself mentally.

•	Web-based features: Remain engaged with different real time features like Netflix, Hulu, or Disney+. Watch motion pictures, Television programs, documentaries, and even pay attention to music, all from the solace of your lounge chair.

•	Online Book shops and Book recordings: Submerge yourself in a decent book with online book shops like Amazon or Barnes and Honorable. Look over an immense choice of digital books or book recordings and appreciate them on your cell phone, tablet, or committed tablet gadget.

Beginning with Innovation:

•	Try not to be threatened! Innovation is intended to be easy to use. Numerous assets are accessible to assist you with getting everything rolling.

•	Request help: Make sure to request for help from your relatives, companions, or even bookkeepers for help with learning new advances.

- Begin little: Pick each or two apparatuses in turn to get to know innovation. You'll be shocked at how rapidly you can get things.

Keep in mind: Innovation is an amazing asset that can improve your life in endless ways. Embrace the potential outcomes, investigate new instruments, and partake in a more associated, helpful, and satisfying life.

Chapter 17
Empowering Yourself: Advocacy and Community Resources for a Fulfilling Golden Age

As a senior citizen, you have a wealth of experience and wisdom to share. You also deserve to have your voice heard and your needs met. This guide will empower you to navigate the world of senior advocacy and connect with valuable community resources, ensuring a fulfilling and engaged golden age.

Understanding Senior Advocacy:

•	What is it? Senior advocacy is the act of promoting and protecting the rights, interests, and well-being of older adults. It involves raising awareness about issues faced by seniors, lobbying for policy changes, and ensuring access to essential resources.

•	Why is it important? Advocacy empowers seniors to have a say in the decisions that affect their lives. It helps ensure access to quality healthcare, affordable housing, and social services.

Getting Involved in Advocacy:

•	Join a Senior Advocacy Organization: Several organizations advocate for senior rights, like AARP (American Association of Retired Persons) or the National Council on Aging. Join their chapters, attend meetings, and participate in advocacy campaigns.

•	Contact Your Elected Officials: Make your voice heard! Contact your local, state, and federal representatives to share your concerns about senior issues. Express your opinions on proposed legislation and advocate for policies that benefit older adults.

•	Speak Up at Public Forums: Public forums offer a platform to share your experiences and advocate for change. Attend town hall meetings, community gatherings, or senior center events, and use your voice to make a difference.

Unveiling a World of Community Resources:

•	Senior Centers: These community hubs offer a variety of programs and services, including social activities, health and wellness workshops, educational courses, and nutritious meals. Many also provide transportation assistance or referrals to other resources.

•	Government Assistance Programs: Several government programs offer financial aid and support services to seniors, such as Social Security, Medicare/Medicaid, and the Supplemental Nutrition Assistance Program (SNAP). Research available programs and don't hesitate to apply for those you qualify for.

•	Volunteer Opportunities: Give back to your community and stay engaged by volunteering your time and skills. Senior centers, local charities, or mentoring programs often welcome the experience and wisdom of older adults.

 Remember: You are not alone! Numerous advocacy organizations and community resources are available to support you. By getting involved, speaking up for your rights, and connecting with the right services, you can ensure a fulfilling, secure, and socially engaged golden age.

Conclusion

Embracing the Gift of Aging – Living A Long, Healthy And Fulfilling Life

Aging is not a decline; it's a transformation. It's a chance to cultivate wisdom, deepen relationships, and embrace new experiences. By prioritizing healthy habits, fostering strong connections, managing stress, and planning for the future, you can turn the golden years into a vibrant chapter filled with purpose, well-being, and a sense of accomplishment.

The tools and resources available today empower you to age well, stay connected, and remain actively engaged in life. Embrace technology, explore your passions, and advocate for your needs. Your voice matters, your experience is valuable, and your journey continues to be an inspiration. So, step forward with confidence, embrace the opportunities that lie ahead, and make the most of the incredible gift of aging.

Acknowledgement

I wish to thank Almighty God for the inspiration to undertake this project and contribute to the society positively.

About the Author

Leo Chambers is a creative writer and Digital Content Creator.

www.ingramcontent.com/pod-product-compliance
Lightning Source LLC
Chambersburg PA
CBHW051817250726
48659CB00005B/1534